The Foundations of Compassion Centered C.A.R.E.

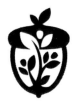

Cheryl Barnes-Neff, PhD, RN

The Foundations of Compassion Centered C.A.R.E.

THE FOUR-STEP PROCESS THAT WILL
CENTER COMPASSION FOR YOU, YOUR TEAM,
AND YOUR PATIENTS

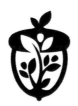

Cheryl Barnes-Neff, PhD, RN

Laurel Oak Press

Table of Contents

Love and compassion are necessities,
not luxuries. Without them,
humanity cannot survive.

~ the Dalai Lama

CHAPTER 1

Why Compassion?

What is compassion, and why is it important in healthcare?

I've seen many patient care models come and go over my forty years as a nurse. From team nursing, to primary care, to care management, all the way to today's most popular model, patient centered care. Patient centered care is certainly a step in the right direction, and has many good points.

I'm proposing that our care model should actually be

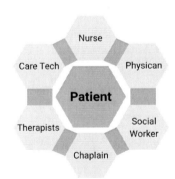

Compassion Centered C.A.R.E. When the patient is in the center of care, the model surrounds the patient with the different disciplines of healthcare professionals, but it implies that we're all doing something *to* the patient, not *with* the patient.

With compassion in the center, we're applying compassion to ourselves, our co-workers, and to our patients and their families. Work moves from being something that expects us to give and give without receiving, to a flow. The current model and systems are not sustainable, despite our herculean efforts to make it work. We exhaust ourselves for

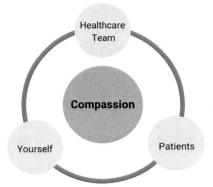

the sake of our patients, but it doesn't have to be that way. Work can also be part of a flow of giving and receiving that nourishes us as we nurture those around us.

While I can't promise that the system will change overnight, I can say that as each of us embrace the idea that compassion can be centered, the model will move toward a more humane way of looking at the work that we do. We will all benefit. Our patients will feel heard and respected for who they are, our co-workers will understand that they are truly part of a team, and we will feel connected to our purpose of a life well lived.

What is Compassion?

There are a number of terms that are used somewhat interchangeably, and that can cause confusion. Words like pity, sympathy, empathy, caring, and compassion are used to describe our feelings when confronted with human suffering. I'd like to propose that we focus on two words: empathy and compassion.

Empathy is the feeling we get when we're touched emotionally by a fellow human who is suffering, and sometimes we not only feel badly that they are suffering, but we can also connect to a feeling within ourselves that resonates. We can never feel exactly the same way another person feels, but we can have a feeling of *Sympatico,* or a feeling of caring and mutual understanding with that person. The problem with empathy is that, while having a empathetic nature is part of what makes life wonderful, it can take us to the brink of empathic distress when we don't know what to do with that feeling.

Compassion includes feelings, but with the added dimension of the intention to act to ease the burden of suffering in the other person. Borrowing from the Buddhist tradition, that desire to act is seen as a response grounded in wisdom within an ethical framework.

What Problems Are We Trying To Solve?

A growing body of research is proving that compassion is more than just "nice to have" in healthcare professionals, it actually saves lives! Compassion is more than "the right thing to do." In the book *Compassionomics*, researchers Stephen Trzeciak and Anthony Mazzerelli spent two years combing through data, studies, and meta analyses discovering that the presence of compassion improved patient outcomes, and just as important, the lack of compassion had devastating consequences.

Does treating patients with compassion really matter?

The answer is far reaching. Compassion matters for patients physiologically, psychologically, socially, and spiritually; motivates self-care and compliance, improves healthcare quality, and improves an organization's bottom line. Oh, and it's an antidote to burnout.

Yet, with all of this goodness, there is a compassion crisis in healthcare. A literal crisis!

You may have read articles recently touting the goodness of compassion and empathy – there's hardly a magazine or website that talks about healthcare that hasn't published an article about empathy and compassion, and how we need more of them. Yet, there is pushback to this idea.

Some of the complaints about the call for more compassion, empathy, and caring in healthcare include: "But, I just don't have time!" "If you care too much, it will break your heart and lead to burnout" and "It doesn't matter what the bedside manner is like, it's if the patient gets out alive that counts." And there's no denying that healthcare has many systemic problems that lead to real challenges in delivering care the way we want to. No one goes into nursing thinking that they will be cold and heartless to people in need, yet when we search our hearts, we've all had days that turned out like that. We make those excuses to keep those days from being more painful than we can bear.

What would it be like if you could come home after your shift – tired for sure – but satisfied that you were able to provide the compassionate care that you would want for your loved ones or for yourself? Care that every patient deserves.

I sincerely believe that staff do care, but sometimes they don't know the best way to provide compassionate care. What are some of the most common problems you're facing?

- ✓ Your staff are frustrated trying to create individualized patient plans of care.
- ✓ Satisfaction surveys coming back low on the "listened and showed respect for the patient" section. Studies show that when that question is answered positively, overall scores are higher.
- ✓ Staff are burned out, not engaged, bullying each other, and generally not happy.
- ✓ You know your staff care, but sometimes they don't know how to be compassionate.
- ✓ You're so frustrated, you're considering going back to the bedside, or leaving nursing all together.

You want your staff to care about each other and your patients. You've tried education and in-services, you may have even tried progressive discipline, or letting staff go to try to turn things around, and nothing seems to work.

The problem is that you've never had a step by stop process to use to teach your staff how to put compassion into action.

CHAPTER 2

Can Compassion Help?

I've made mistakes working with patients, and have gone home in tears because I couldn't give the care I wanted to give. I was told that I had to harden my heart to my patients' pain or I wouldn't make it. There were times that I took that advice, wanting to be an ICU badass: clinical all the way through. But then, a patient or a patient's family would pierce my heart with their pain – pain that came from the depth of their love.

Once, when I was waiting in the lobby for a friend that was having a minor procedure done, a surgeon came out to find a patient's family, calling "Loved ones! I'm looking for the loved ones of Mrs. Smith." I just loved that! I started referring to my patient's "loved ones" ever since.

Compassion in healthcare has been part of my professional and personal journey throughout my life.

The Coronavirus crisis has brought the need for compassion into sharp relief. Personally, I think this is a water-shed moment for all of us. On the site *"Dear World,"* nurses have been telling their stories of becoming more aware of the need for compassion than ever before. A nurse named Sarah Wells told her story of having the "hardened shell" around her heart broken. She explains about her patient:

"This day was her last and she was spoken to mostly through a glass door or by people garbed up - she didn't even know what her caregivers looked like. How terrifying. Losing a patient is never easy, but the nature of caring for trauma patients has a way of hardening you.

This day, the hardened shell I had built completely shattered and the tears were plentiful. Those around me commented, 'What's wrong with you? We do this every day!' I felt the same way, but I couldn't control it."[1]

My guess is that you've had a similar experience – I know I have. And on those days, we have an important choice to make. To allow that shell to be forever shattered,

---

[1] #DearNurses. *Dear World.org*. https://nurses.dearworld.org/013-I-ve-Never-Cried-Like-That-About-A-Patient-1

and bring compassion into all of our care, or to stay co-cooned by pain.

For decades now, I've been working on the problem of what compassionate care looks like. Starting in the Neona-tal Intensive Care Unit, and working my way to hospice as both a nurse and chaplain, I've trained new nurses, chap-lains and social workers, and volunteers on how they can bring their compassion into the world.

Lots of the suggestions you'll read if you do a search on "How is compassion shown in nursing?" will include things like making eye contact, treating the patient with kindness, holding their hand, and giving them your full at-tention. All of those things are good, but they don't go far enough.

I've developed a four-step process to be applied to your-self, your co-workers and staff, and to your patients and their families.

The C.A.R.E. Process

One of the hallmarks of compassionate care is often re-ferred to as simply being the Golden Rule: Do unto others as you would have them do unto you. The problem comes in when we start working with the wide variety of patients and their families, and our co-workers. We live in a plural-istic society, and even in groups that seem to be pretty much the same, there is a wide array of opinions and preferences.

Better might be called the Platinum Rule: Treat others the way they want to be treated. In other words, we have to ask them to know how they want to be treated. The C.A.R.E. process will lead you and your staff through finding out what is important to the patient through responding to them with dignity and respect, the heart of compassion.

Here's how it works: C.A.R.E. is an acronym for Connect, Assess, Respond, and Evaluate and End the encounter. These are steps you can implement right now to improve your life as a nurse leader, increase staff engagement and performance, and improve the satisfaction of your patients.

It's applied first to yourself. It's important that you understand the process on a personal level, and for you to exemplify the process to your staff and patients. This can't be a "do as I say, not as I do" kind of thing!

It's next applied to your staff and co-workers. Understanding your staff, and helping them understand each other will help in your efforts for improved communication, respectful behavior, and engagement and morale.

Finally, it's applied to your patients and their families. When the staff sees you listening to them, it's a light bulb effect, and they naturally take that ideal of listening to their patients. Let's look at each step.

Connect

Connection is what human beings need, thrive on, and long for. When we connect with others, we feel a sense of security, trust, being understood, and belonging. Connecting to ourselves might sound a bit strange at first, but the simple act of taking a breath – from the tip of our nose, to the tips of our toes – reconnects us to our bodies and is instantly refreshing.

Connecting to our staff helps to build team work, and helps them feel heard, and understood. Our patients, too, need that feeling of connection to feel safe. They come to us feeling uncertain, and even terrified. Simply making eye contact with a smile can be the beginning of building the trusting relationship they need on their path to recovery.

Assess

Assessment is what nurses do best, and we're going to take our assessment skills to the next level. When we assess our patients, we are really good at recognizing and understanding their bodily structures and functions. We use charting checklists that guide us through a head-to-toe systems review. What is sometimes missing are patient preferences, their social determinants of health, and the support they need. This sounds like a tall order, but it actually boils down to asking a single question: "What matters to you?"

There are many uses for this simple question, both to better understand our patients – to know who they are as people – as well as better understanding our staff and coworkers. When staff feel heard, they can express the underlying reasons for how they react to the things that upset them. When they feel heard, they feel more connected and part of a team.

When we assess ourselves, we not only ask ourselves "What matters to me?" but we can also take time to explore our assumptions about ourselves, our staff, and our patients. We need to ask "Is that true?" or "Am I sure?" and interrogate that assumption. We might find that when we get curious, when we start listening to their story, we make more room for empathy and compassion. One of my favorite quotes of Mr. Rogers is:

> *"Frankly, there isn't anyone you couldn't learn to love once you've heard their story."*

Which leads to Respond

When we react to a situation, we often say or do things we later regret. We might feel the reaction is justified, but when we look back, we have that feeling that we wish we had done things differently.

I've been there – more than once.

But we can learn to respond instead of react. Let's add "respond with respect" to the mix as well. When we know the person's story, we still might not agree with their choices or decisions, but we do get a little closer to understanding why they are the way they are. We get to know them as person.

When we do that, we can get a lot closer to giving them the best possible care. Remember our analogy above about the Platinum Rule? The people we care for are unique individuals, so when it comes time to provide care, communicate with them, or connect with them, it needs to be on their terms. Then the compassionate action becomes action that will actually serve them; not just a canned checkmark on a list of interventions.

This becomes the individualized plan of care. A discharge plan the patient can actually follow.

Did a lightbulb just go off? I know, right?

Evaluate and End the Encounter

No nursing process would be complete without spending a moment on evaluating the interaction. Did our interventions work? We can also add looking at how well we were able to connect with our patients, were we able to assess their situation honestly, and respond to them with compassion?

Applying this to ourselves and our staff is also important. Having an end of shift checklist for ourselves can be enlightening and helpful. Not as a way to beat ourselves up, but to look at the progress we're making, and if this method is working.

In Joan Halifax's book *Standing at the Edge*, she offers sage advice for engaging with the suffering we see all around us with integrity. While I've developed and used my C.A.R.E. model over the past decades of work, I was inspired by Roshi Joan's addition of *End* to the process. She says, "When the time is right, we mark the end of our time… so that we can move cleanly to the next moment, person, or task." She goes on to say, "Without the acknowledgment of what has taken place, it can be difficult to let go of this encounter and move on." This is so important.

Have you ever found that you wake up at 3 in the morning worrying (or is it just me?), or that you spend time worrying about work when you're home, only to turn around and worry about home while you're at work?

Having a definitive *End* to our interactions and encounters goes a long way to solve this problem, bring peace of mind to our lives.

I've been working in the hospice field for the past twenty years, and one of the things I learned early on was to say goodbye to my patients at the end of every visit. Even if it was just to make eye contact, and hold their hand with a smile. The reality is that we might not see that patient again.

We might have a little ritual of being sure we at least wave bye to each of our staff at the end of the shift, touch base with anyone who needs help to finish, and to have our own "goodbye" before leaving the floor. Even something as simple as taking off our lanyard, hanging it in our locker, and saying "see you tomorrow."

CHAPTER 3

The C.A.R.E. Process

Let's take a closer look, not only at how important compassion is to care, but also at a practical step-by-step process to make it easy to take action on the compassion you feel for your patients. Compassion is a hallmark of patient care. Yet many would say that empathy and compassion are in short supply today.

Studies show that compassion is not a luxury, but a necessity to improve patient outcomes and satisfaction, reduce staff burnout, and even impact revenue in a positive way. This book will introduce the four-step process C.A.R.E. as a way to practice and teach compassion. This will enable you to: Describe the importance of empathy and compassion in patient care, identify the component steps in the C.A.R.E. process, list who the C.A.R.E. process applies to, and describe how to evaluate improvements to practice patterns and outcomes after implementing the methodology.

Because we know that studies show the importance of compassion care for patients, it's crucial that we train healthcare professionals in compassionate care. Patients are affected physiologically, psychologically, socially and spiritually by compassionate care, so all disciplines must be involved. All disciplines can act within their scope of practice in a compassionate way.

There are a number of problems we are proposing can be solved with the application of effective, appropriate compassionate care. If you're a nurse leader, you might find that your staff are struggling with creating individualized plans of care, satisfaction surveys are coming back low on the listened and showed respect for the patient section, or patients are unable to follow their discharge plans. Staff are burned out, not engaged, bullying each other, and generally not happy. Staff morale makes a big difference in the effectiveness of the care provided. When staff don't feel that they are being treated with dignity and respect – or with compassion – their satisfaction in their work suffers, and this can take many forms.

You know your staff care, but sometimes they don't know how to be compassionate. We mentioned earlier that there have been many recent articles in healthcare journals about empathy, compassion, and self-care.

Yet, for many healthcare professionals burdened with short staffing, low pay, and a system that doesn't treat them with respect, it's not surprising to hear some nurses complain that empathy, compassion, and self-care are not going to solve the over-all problems. And they're right! There's no denying that healthcare has many systemic problems that lead to real challenges in delivering care the way we want to. It seems like many of the efforts encouraging self care, empathy, and compassion are merely Band-Aids for these serious problems. And, even worse blaming the victim!

Yoga class won't fix the healthcare system, and any nostalgia for the "good old days" is just that – nostalgia. There have always been systemic problems preventing true compassion centered care. We can't go back. We need to design our work life with compassion at the center so we can move forward in a way that is sustainable and nourishing to everyone involved.

It is important to treat ourselves, our co-workers, and our patients with compassion. No one goes into nursing thinking they will be cold and heartless to people in need. Yet, it does seem that there are some unit cultures that foster a cynical approach to patients with little empathy, and it seems that there are many excuses for that behavior. It can be different. What would it be like if you could come home after your shift, tired for sure, but satisfied that you were able to provide the compassionate care that you would want for your loved ones or for yourself; care that every patient deserves?

So how do you mandate compassion? You can't! But you can turn things around. Why haven't other approaches worked? The problem is you've never had a process to use step-by-step to use and to teach your staff how to put compassion into action.

I've heard many lectures with thought leaders in the healthcare, spiritual, and secular mindfulness field teach about how to become more compassionate. They tend to focus on the feelings of compassion, and how to cultivate those feelings in a healthy way. Those programs are very valuable, and all of us can use programs to help us be more in touch with our heart. However, what is missing – and what I often hear nurses ask in the Q&A sessions is: *How* do we act on the compassion we feel? We've had many experiences of feeling empathy, reaching out with compassion, only to be frustrated that nothing seemed to work. The person didn't understand our motivation, and might even have been offended, or we couldn't get past their disrespectful or combative behavior.

Like you, I became a nurse leader because I saw areas in my unit that needed improvement, and I knew that through staff education and modeling quality care, I could make a difference. But, what I found is that simply telling someone what to do doesn't work. We just can't tell our staff "Be more compassionate!" They may well come back with "I *am* compassionate! Show me what to do about it!"

We have to show them and teach them specifics. We nurses tend to be "bottom liners."

We want a formula:
- ✓ What's the problem?
- ✓ What's the rationale?
- ✓ What do I need to do?
- ✓ How do I document this?

As a nurse leader you want to know:
- ✓ What is the ideal practice?
- ✓ What are the gaps in knowledge and practice?
- ✓ What are the steps to implement the change?
- ✓ How will I know that it's working?

But, let's back up a bit and talk about compassion, what it is and why it's important in healthcare. There are a number of terms that can be used somewhat interchangeably that can cause confusion. Words like pity, sympathy, empathy, caring, and compassion are used to describe our feelings when confronted with human suffering.

The following is an excerpt from an animated talk by Brené Brown, researcher and social worker, talking about the distinction between empathy and sympathy:

"So what is empathy, and why is it very different than sympathy? Empathy fuels connection. Sympathy drives disconnection... Teresa Wiseman is a nursing scholar who studied professions – very diverse professions – where empathy is relevant and came up with four qualities of empathy:

- Perspective taking - the ability to take the perspective of another person or recognize their perspective as their truth,
- Staying out of judgement – not easy when you enjoy it as much as most of us do,
- Recognizing emotion in other people,
- And then communicating that.

"Empathy is feeling with people. And to me, I always think of empathy as this kind of sacred space when someone is kind of in a deep hole, and they shout out from the bottom and they say, 'I'm stuck. It's dark. I'm overwhelmed.' And then we look and we say, 'Hey, I know what it's like down here, and you're not alone'...

"Empathy is a choice, and it's a vulnerable choice. Because in order to connect with you, I have to connect with something in myself that knows that feeling. Rarely, if ever, does an empathic response begin with 'at least.'... But one of the things we do sometimes in the face of very difficult conversations is we try to make things better. If I share something you that's very difficult, I'd rather you say I don't even know what to say right now. I'm *just so glad you told me. Because the truth is rarely can a re-sponse make something better. What makes something better is connection."[2]*

The Vocabulary of Caring

Empathy is a feeling we get when we're touched emotionally by a fellow human who is suffering. And sometimes we not only feel badly that they're suffering, but can also connect to a feeling within ourselves that resonates. We can never feel exactly the same way another person feels, but we can have a feeling of *Sympatico* or a feeling of caring and mutual understanding with that person. The problem with empathy is that while having an empathic nature is part of what makes life wonderful, it can take us to the brink of empathic distress when we don't know what to do with that feeling.

Compassion includes feelings, but with the added dimension of the intention to act; to ease the burden of suffering in the other person. It's also important that the compassionate responses are grounded in wisdom, discernment, and an ethical framework.

---

[2] Please watch the video: Brown, Brené. (2013) *Brené Brown on Empathy*. The RSA. https://youtu.be/1Evwgu369Jw

We heard in the video that nursing scholar Theresa Wiseman has suggested that there are four main attributes of empathy. They are:

- Perspective taking,
- Staying out of judgment,
- Recognizing emotions in others, and
- Communicating back the emotion you see.

Brené Brown says that empathy fuels connection, and that empathy is a choice. And, as she says, "…it's a vulnerable choice because in order to connect with you, I have to connect with something in myself that knows that feeling."

We try our best to stay out of judgment, but that can be tough. We've all heard phrases like, "Oh, that's silly, who would get upset about that?" or "I've been through that and I didn't have a meltdown," or "It could be worse!" You might not say these kinds of things to the person, but having these feelings does color the way we respond to them.

Staying out of judgment, though, doesn't mean to ignore or bottle our feelings about our judgements. We need to own our judgements. I was giving a talk about this idea to a group, and before I could say more about that, a participant gave me a thumbs up – "that's right!" Now, I think she had jumped the gun a bit and might have thought I was saying we should celebrate our judgements, and that's not what I mean at all! When we see that we have a judgement, it's important to ask ourselves "Is that true?" or "Am I sure?" We want to stay in alignment with our values, for sure, but when we're judging someone to be "too sensitive," or having a "chip on their shoulder," or whatever other negative trait we believe they have, we should question that – even if, maybe especially if, it makes us uncomfortable. We may well find that when we work with a patient and their family without an agenda, they feel they can open up to us and when we get to know them better, we can understand their world view.

This can be tough because we've also spent a great deal of time, effort, and commitment to learn the best treatments and solutions to our patient's medical problems. It's easy to feel that they're not trying hard enough, or if only they would make better life choices, they wouldn't be in the situation they're in. We might even wonder aloud, "why did they come to the hospital if they didn't want the treatments we provide?" When we can recognize our feel ings of judgment and interrogate them within ourselves, we may find that we can have more empathy for our patients by recognizing the social, cultural, financial, and systemic determinants that affect their worldview.

Compassion includes feelings, but with the added dimension of the intention to act, to ease the burden of suffering in the other effectively and within an ethical framework.

Is There a Difference?

So let's take a closer look at the many words that are used to describe how we feel about the situations of others. Is there a difference between them, and does it really matter which words we use? We have many feelings that we experience within ourselves our family our friends and community, as well as our co-workers and patients.

Empathy can take the form of:

- Empathic concern,
- Cognitive empathy, and
- Emotional empathy.

Emotional empathy is feeling with the other person and is an important part of our connection and relationship with others. Cognitive empathy is understanding how people see and think about the world. We can understand that a person would be very upset, fearful, happy, sad, and more by recognizing that their perspective and feelings are true for them. Having empathic concern creates a foundation for our nursing practice. We create a caring environment for the people around us.

It's really not reasonable or healthy to expect a healthcare professional to experience emotional empathy with each and every patient. Yet we can have cognitive empathy, meaning that we take the other person's perspective and imagine what it would be like to be in their situation.

By having a strong foundation of empathic concern, we can approach the other person with caring and compassion. What we do want to guard against is the experience of empathic distress.

As nurses, we want to help our patients and fix what ails them. In other words, we're altruistic. But if we over identify with our patient's pain and suffering, we can begin to feel burned out. We're suffering from empathic distress, the repeated exposure to the trauma of others. Compassion on the other hand, reveals the best course of action to take to help a person within their worldview. It's a feeling of caring, but also a desire to help. And what we'll see as a way to take action that not only helps the other person, but helps us as well. Compassion is being present with our patients and truly listening to them. The step-by-step framework C.A.R.E., will show you how to do this.

We'll see how the C.A.R.E. Framework will make your care more effective.

The goal is always to help our patients by easing the burden of their suffering, and partnering with them for the best possible care and support.

You'll find that this framework is also very satisfying for you as a nurse or other healthcare professional. By listening to our patients in an objective and nonjudgmental way, we can release the stress that we sometimes feel when we believe we must give the patient the one right plan. And if that plan isn't followed, we've somehow failed. By creatively and open-heartedly trusting our patients to know what's best for them at any given time, we can treat them with respect, and then they feel that they can trust us. Listening builds trust, and trust builds confidence. Patients can then accept and take our best advice, especially when that advice takes their needs and their values into account. Now let's look at the practical step-by-step way to put this into action: C.A.R.E.

The Steps of C.A.R.E.

We've mentioned the Golden Rule: "Do unto others, as you would have them do unto you." For many of us, that seems like the best place to start. The problem comes in when we start working with a wide variety of patients and their families, and even our co-workers. We live in a pluralistic society. Even in groups that seem to be pretty much the same, there is a wide array and variety of opinions and preferences. And, honestly, even if we live in a place where everyone seems pretty much the same, each person you meet wants to be treated as an individual – not so different from any other place in the world.

Better might be called the Platinum Rule: "Treat others the way they want to be treated." To do that, we have to ask them to know how they want to be treated. The C.A.R.E. process will lead you and your staff through finding out what is important to the patient, then responding to them with dignity and respect: The heart of compassion.

The steps of C.A.R.E. are Connect, Assess, Respond, and Evaluate and End the encounter. They are steps that you can implement right now to improve your life as a nurse leader, see increased staff engagement and performance, and improve the satisfaction of your patients.

Who are the steps applied to?

The steps are applied first to yourself. It's important that you understand the process on a personal level and for you to exemplify the process to your co-workers, staff and patients. This can't be a "Do as I say, not as I do" kind of thing. This is going beyond self-care, and while bubble baths and yoga are nice – keep doing that if you enjoy it – you'll be learning ways to develop self compassion that go beyond quick fixes.

It's next applied to your staff and co-workers, understanding your staff and helping them understand each other will help in your efforts for improved teamwork, communication, engagement, and morale.

Finally, it's applied to your patients and their families. As a nurse leader, when the staff sees you listening to them, it's a light bulb effect. They naturally take that ideal of listening to their patients in turn.

We'll learn the importance of asking "What matters to you?" as a good start to understanding and listening to our patients so that we can give them the best possible care.

Let's Look At The Action Steps: How to C.A.R.E.

Connections matter. When we have human connection, we feel a sense of security, trust, being understood, and belonging. A sense of social connection is one of our fundamental human needs. Without it, we can actually get sick. Psychologist Emma Seppälä says that social connections generate a positive feedback loop of social, emotional, and physical wellbeing. Unfortunately, the opposite is also true for those who lack social connections. Low social connection has been generally associated with declines in physical and psychological health, as well as a higher propensity to antisocial behavior leading to further isolation.

The first step in C.A.R.E. is Connect, and the first person we need to apply this step to is ourselves. Taking centering or cleansing breaths helps us listen to our body and emotions. It starts the process of self compassion.

Connecting to our staff and co-workers helps build teamwork and helps them feel heard and understood. Using active listening means we can learn what's important to them. Our patients, too, need that feeling of connection to feel safe. They come to us feeling uncertain, even terri-fied. Simply making eye contact with a smile can be the be-ginning of building that trusting relationship they need on their path to recovery. We want to ask what matters to them; what we need to know about them as a person to take the best possible care of them. To listen and to under-stand.

The second step is Assess. It starts with ourselves, and is an important consideration for our co-workers, and our patients. When we can get in touch with our feelings, know our personal values, and recognize our feelings it helps us understand ourselves better. Assessment is valuable for working with our team. You probably have a good work friend that you can tell at a glance if they're having a bad day and it's best to leave them be, or when they need a helping hand.

As a nurse leader, and all nurses are leaders, it's im-portant to assess a situation with your staff without judg-ment; as objectively as possible. You don't want to jump to conclusions and wind up saying something you'll regret.

For patients, doing an assessment is what nurses do best. We're going to take our assessment skills to the next level. When we assess our patients, we're really good at recognizing and understanding their bodily structures and functions. We use charting checklists that guide us through head to toe systems review.

What is sometimes missing though, are patient preferences, their social determinants of health, and the support they need. This sounds like a tall order, but it actually boils down to asking a single question. "What matters to you?" There are many uses for this simple question, both to better understand our patients, to know who they are as people, as well as better understanding our staff and co-workers.

We might find out that when we get curious and when we start listening to their story, we make more room for empathy and compassion. And when we make that room and act on it, we often find that we benefit as well. Fred Rogers explains:

"All of us, at some time or other, need help. Whether we're giving or receiving help, each one of us has something valuable to bring to this world. That's one of the things that connects us as neighbors-- in our own way, each one of us is a giver and a receiver."

The "R" in C.A.R.E. stands for Respond. We want to respond instead of react, and we always want to respond with respect. When we react to a situation we often say or do things we later regret, we might feel that reaction is justified. But when we look back, we have that feeling that we wish we'd done things differently. I've been there - more than once.

So instead of a knee-jerk reaction, we want to respond. Listen carefully. Take a pause when you're feeling reactive, and decide how best to approach the situation. We can learn to respond with respect instead of reacting. When we know the person's story, we still might not agree with their choices or decisions, but we do get a little closer to understanding why they are the way they are. We get to know them as a person.

When we do that, we can get a lot closer to giving them the best possible care. Remember our analogy about the Platinum Rule? The people we care for are unique individuals. So when it comes time to provide care, communicate with them or connect with them, it needs to be on their terms. Then the compassionate action becomes action that will actually serve them, not just to add a check mark on a list of interventions. This becomes the individualized plan of care and a discharge plan the patient can actually follow.

The "E" stands for Evaluate and End. No nursing process would be complete without spending a moment evaluating the interaction. Did our interventions work? When reviewing the care plan, we evaluate how well the interventions worked, adjust our responses accordingly, and modify the plan. We can apply this to ourselves, and our staff as well.

Having an end of shift checklist for ourselves can be enlightening and helpful, not as a way to beat ourselves up, but to look at the progress we're making. Were we able to assess their situation honestly, and respond to them with compassion?

In Joan Halifax's book, *Standing at the Edge*, she offers sage advice for engaging with the suffering that we see all around us with integrity. She says when the time is right, we mark the end of our time so that we can move cleanly to the next moment person or task. She goes on to explain that without the acknowledgement of what has taken place, it can be difficult to let go of this encounter and move on.

We might have a little ritual of being sure that we at least wave goodbye to each of our staff at the end of the shift, touch base with anyone who needs help to finish, and then have our own goodbye before leaving the floor. Even something as simple as taking off our lanyard, hanging it in our locker and saying, "see you tomorrow."

CHAPTER 4

Who C.A.R.E. Applies To

C.A.R.E. About You

Now, let's take a deeper dive into the steps of C.A.R.E. as they apply to ourselves.

C.A.R.E. for yourself is the first step. It's important that you understand the process on a personal level, and for you to exemplify the process to your staff and patients. As we said before, this can't be a "do as I say, not as I do!" kind of thing.

Connect

The first step in C.A.R.E. is Connect. And the first person we apply this step to is ourselves. As we said, connecting to ourselves might seem strange at first, but the simple act of taking a breath, reconnects us to our bodies and is instantly refreshing. Taking centering breaths, helps us to listen to our bodies and emotions. Even on our busiest day, we can take a deep breath. Have you ever said "I was so busy I didn't even have time to breathe"? That saying is a good reminder of the importance of breathing.

When we wash our hands or use hand sanitizer, we can use those precious seconds to breathe and simply focus on our hands. You might look at your hands and have a feeling of gratitude for the work of your hands.

Placing your hand on your heart can be a way to get back in touch with your body, your feelings, and your spirit. Deborah Grassman of the Opus Peace Project recommends this in order to ground ourselves, especially when we're tempted to say "I'm beside myself!" This helps when we're in need of courage, strength, or patience.

Connecting to ourselves takes practice, and an ongoing practice of meditation, contemplative prayer, or secular mindfulness can be very helpful.

Assess to Know Yourself

To focus and enhance our personal self-awareness, Assess starts with ourselves, too. We might be tempted to think that assessment means finding what's wrong, but our goal here is to see ourselves as we really are.

It's important to know our strengths, as well as those aspects that need improvement. We want to understand ourselves better. When we ask "What matters to me?" this can be as simple and fun as saying, playing with my dog to something as important as my family and my faith. Knowing what matters helps to guide us in the way we live our lives. In addition, making a list of our values is important as an internal compass that keeps us pointing in the right direction. Your values are your personal truth, and when you keep your values in mind, you're acting from your values rather than what others think you should or ought to do.

Taking a close look at your emotions helps develop flexibility and resilience. When we realize that we *have* emotions; that we are not our emotions, we can understand that emotions aren't demands to action.

Knowing our authentic identity helps us ensure that our actions come from a place of honesty. We have many identities and roles in our lives. Things like "I'm a nurse," "I'm a mother or father, son, daughter," "I'm proud of my Italian heritage and make fantastic tomato sauce," and many more. Be aware of the identity messages that are disparaging like "I'm no good," "I'm stupid," or other negative self-talk. Make sure that you treat yourself as well as you would treat a good friend.

As a nurse leader, you can also assess your leadership style and communication skills. By working on those skills, you can enhance your team's success.

Respond with Respect

How we respond to situations is the key to interactions with others. We want to Respond instead of reacting out of emotion, frustration, or a sense of payback for behavior we feel is inappropriate. Responding is what happens to us is a sign of emotional intelligence.

We're connecting with ourselves when we notice that we're feeling emotional or triggered. We assess that we have the emotion, but we are not that emotion. When we can take time to pause and realize this, we're more likely to respond in alignment with our values.

We always want to respond with respect. You may have heard others say, or maybe have said yourself: "Respect is earned," or "I'll treat them with respect when they treat me with respect!" However, especially in a professional environment, taking the high road and treating everyone with respect allows us to act in a way that is compassionate. Along with this, using the Platinum Rule and treating others the way they want to be treated, can make responses more meaningful and effective. When we take the worldview of the other person into account, communication is more successful.

Evaluation

We all have our off days. And even with the best of intentions, we might want to say something we know we'll regret. Now I know how satisfying saying that zinger out loud can feel in the moment – we won't talk about why I know that – but trust me, that satisfied moment passes into regret pretty quickly. Take a breather if you possibly can, and let the person know that now is not the time for a discussion.

Evaluate: The nursing process wouldn't be complete without evaluating the patient's response to a treatment or medication. And the same is true for our efforts in interacting and communicating with others during the day. Evaluate your assessments of situations, and your responses. Not with an eye to be critical or find all that went wrong, but by looking at what worked and what didn't. If you've ever played a sport, you know that your coach is there to help guide you to the best possible performance. You want to hear even the most minute detail because of your desire to learn the skill and excel. Understand that these are skills and we need practice to improve. Consider yourself your personal encouraging, very best possible coach – one that will draw your attention to things that can be improved.

An Attitude of Gratitude

In that evaluation, it's important to embrace gratitude. Look for at least three things that went right, that you saw from others, or that you found along the way that were good. It might be something as simple as a flower arrangement in a patient's room, or maybe as you were walking in from the parking lot a bright red cardinal perched in a tree, and it looked really beautiful against the blue sky. Maybe you calmed a patient, and they got some much needed sleep, or you saw one of your staff give a co-worker a well-deserved "atta girl." All of those things are cause for feeling grateful. Last but not least, bring an end to your shift, and leave work behind peacefully.

Ending

Have you ever spent a shift at work worried about what was going on at home, but once you got home, found yourself worrying about what was going on at work? A better way is to end not only the shift, but each encounter we find ourselves in. We can relieve a lot of stress by doing our best in each encounter, then letting the situation go and moving on to the next situation.

This is different from compartmentalizing. Compartmentalization of our feelings is actually a defense mechanism we use to protect us from cognitive dissonance. Now, while I've heard so-called life hackers talk about the bene-fits of compartmentalizing, separating our feelings into boxes or bottling our feelings might seem like a good idea and might even be helpful in the short term, but it can re-ally be harmful in the long run.

One of our goals is to be an authentic person who lives by our values, and can see the big picture of any situation. Compartmentalizing our thoughts and feelings, narrow our thinking. Instead, we want to bring our values and best selves to each interaction with others. We do that by being fully present to the situation.

Yet when the interaction is over, we can remind our-selves that it's time to let go of the situation, and go on to the next interaction fully, not taking anxiety and stress along with us. At the end of the shift, we could use a check-list that reminds us that we can trust our co-workers to take good care of our patients. We can recall good things that happen during the shift. Touch base with co-workers, to be sure they're okay or if they need help finishing; say good-bye to patients as appropriate.

And now it's time to focus on our family, friends, pets, or our own quiet time, and be at home wholeheartedly.

C.A.R.E. About Your Team

C.A.R.E. is next applied to staff and co-workers, under-standing your team and helping them understand each other will help in your efforts for improved teamwork, communication, engagement, and morale.

Connection

To connect with your staff and co-workers is very important when we're busy during the day. Sometimes we can forget to connect with our co-workers, but it's important that we connect throughout the day and are honest in how we're doing. Check in with co-workers to see if they need a hand and be willing to ask for help. Sometimes we act like the lone ranger thinking we'll be valued for being able to do it all ourselves. The reality is that we're part of a team, and we need good team building skills.

Listening Skills

Active listening is important, too. We need to do our best not to interrupt our co-workers. When they're explaining something, we might believe we already know the rest. So why do we have to listen to the whole thing? And I think we all realize that it's pretty rude to do that. When we give someone our undivided attention, they feel respected and valued.

We can ask "What matters to you?" of each other as well. If you're a nurse leader, you could consider asking that question during a team meeting and listening to the answers, getting to know each other on a meaningful level. It's important to be aware of our co-workers' background, family situations, culture, and worldview. We do need to be mindful in our approach to learning these aspects of our co-workers lives. While we want to be aware of who they are as people, we also want to be respectful and not cross any personal boundaries.

As a nurse leader, an important part of your role is to assess your staff. You may have a formal process and forms to fill out to complete an employee performance appraisal. You'll be observing your staff on a regular basis to assess their job performance, communication skills, ability to work with the team, and setting goals for the coming year. Be sure that you're examining your opinions about staff members to assure that you're not taking someone else's opinion, or have come to a snap judgment based on a single observation.

It's important to keep a sense of balance as you observe your staff. Be sure to look just as carefully at their strengths as their weaknesses. Giving praise and encouragement at the time these positive actions occur, is a good way to build a positive work environment for everyone, even when improvement is needed. When staff feel that they're being coached because you want the best for them, and that you see their potential, the result is beneficial for everyone. What are their coping skills responses? Do they tend to be reactive or have some bad habits in their communication with others? Sometimes people don't realize that they're coming across as snippy, grouchy, or rude, or it could be that their co-workers aren't understanding a cultural response to situations. However, if you see signs of incivility or even bullying, be prepared to take action as soon as possible. Meet with a staff member privately and let them know that professional behavior is expected, and disruptive behavior will not be tolerated.

Respond and Communication

Communication is a two-way street. So be sure to notice what's happening with the staff member as you're interacting, especially if it's a difficult conversation. Sometimes we believe that we can size someone up and make a judgment about them at a glance. We think we're fantastic judges of human nature just by looking. In reality, that's just not the case. It's important not to give ourselves credit for good judgment of human nature, when it's actually an unconscious bias. The other person might be closed off and might not like us at first glance either, but it's often baggage from interactions with other people. Maybe we remind them of their Aunt Gertrude who was mean to them when they were a kid.

Respond instead of react, and stay civil and respectful so we don't add fuel to that unnecessary fire. It's important to clear up misunderstandings promptly and not perpetuate the vicious cycle of labeling them as having a chip on their shoulder, or having a character flaw.

Conflict Resolution

Having a method for conflict resolution is important to keep the lines of communication open, and resolve problems before they take on a life of their own. Remember that there will be times that problems may arise that you, as a frontline nurse manager, have no control over. There may be staffing shortages, poor communication from administration, and systems that are, frankly, unfair that everyone has to deal with. Be honest with your staff about what you can and cannot control, and how you've taken their concerns to management. You'll be able to update them on any policy changes that may affect them. Be sure that they know that you're on their side, and that your team can work together to make it through tough times. Strive to build consensus and give staff as much control as possible for decision making. If you're responsible for the staffing calendar, you might consider involving staff members in this shared task, or contributing to the criteria for making assignments. Being transparent in how decisions are made, and assuring the decisions are as fair as possible, goes a long way toward positive staff morale.

Leadership Skills

Showing genuine interest in each other, and getting to know each other as people builds teamwork. Taking the teams' temperature regularly prevents minor issues from becoming more serious.

By taking the team's temperature. I mean that it's good to come up with ideas for checking on staff regularly. This may take the form of a morning huddle. Or, it might mean checking in with each person on the floor, jumping in to help with the dressing change, turning a patient, doing a bath, or whatever is needed. You can observe the care given, demonstrate best practices, or simply touch base to see if everything is going well for that staff person.

The goal is for staff to feel heard and understood. If you're the frontline nurse leader, it can be a challenge to seek out and touch base with each staff member with all the other work you're responsible for, but it's worth the effort. And it will make a big difference!

If you're not the frontline nurse leader. That doesn't mean that nothing can be done. You can make the effort to contribute to a positive team environment, being sure that you don't join in gossip or other disruptive behavior, and keep a positive attitude. Getting to know your co-workers can make a big difference in everyone's work life.

When staff morale is low, nurse leaders should take immediate action to look at the quality of care. Quality is directly related to staff morale, and evaluating the quality of care delivered and patient outcomes will also point you in the direction of staff problems. Data-driven solutions can improve patient outcomes, staff satisfaction, and pride for the team.

Remember, studies show that staff don't quit the organization, they quit the manager. By keeping the lines of communication open, the staff will see that you're on their side. When we're engaged, our work has meaning, and we feel energized and alive. We'll go home tired for sure, but it's a good tired when we've made a difference. Without meaning our tiredness makes us bone weary.

C.A.R.E. for Our Patients

Let's take a look at the steps of C.A.R.E. applied to patient care. The process allows us to recognize our patients as individuals with their own priorities, preferences, and choices.

Connect

Connections matter. When we have human connection, we feel a sense of security, trust, being understood, and belonging. Connect with your patients by establishing rapport. Call them by their preferred name, pronouns, et cetera. Connecting with patients is a crucial part of the patient's feeling of confidence that they will be cared for. They're often frightened and anxious about what is happening, and may feel no one truly cares about them. Everything we do and say makes an impact on them. So we must be careful not to cause them more anxiety and concern.

To make a connection, we can make eye contact, shake hands if appropriate, and make sure we call them by the correct name, pronouns, and have a caring stance.

In some cultures, being smiley and cheerful when they are sick and worried might seem insensitive. A smile and a fleeting touch can telegraph a feeling of care, and studies show that "grammy-grandpa" talk harms patients. You've probably heard staff talk with an elder in that kind of, "How are we doing today, Pops?" or, "Oh, you're so cute!" as they pat the patient on the head. Patients with dementia are less cooperative and more combative when spoken to as though they are children. Instead, call each patient by the name may prefer. For some, that name may be a different than the one that's on their medical record. We want to be sure to balance patient safety for identification, treatments, and medication administration, while honoring the patient's priorities around their name and identity.

For elders, it's best to call them by their surname and last name. They may say it's okay to call them by a nickname, but until you've known them for awhile, err on the side of honor and respect.

Be sure to remember consent. Ask permission to touch, and be sure to describe what's going on in detail, and what will be done to the patient step-by-step. Understand cultural aspects of personal contact, and have cultural humility. Don't assume you know, be sure to ask.

Assess

Assess your patient and their family. In addition to head to toe assessment ask: "What matters to you?" Listen to the answers, learn what their healthcare priorities are, and learn about their culture, family dynamics, and home life. The answers are the basis of what we should do for them.

To understand our patients, we need to know who they are as people. We want to know what is wrong with the patient and what concerns have brought to them to us for care, of course, but we also want to know what matters to them as people. We can ask a number of questions to find out more about their priorities, what social determinants of health are present that might affect their care, and what their support needs are. It's important to know what family, culture, religion, social situation, and other aspects might impact their life. We might find that when we get curious, when we start listening to their story, we make more room for empathy and compassion. As I said earlier, one of my favorite quotes of Mr. Rogers is: "Frankly, there isn't anyone you couldn't learn to love once you've heard their story."

Listening Skills

We like to think of ourselves as good listeners, but it's important to take a closer look at our listening skills. Listening is a key component of assessment. We need to discover the patient's history, their chief complaints, and their observations and reports about their symptoms. There are a number of types of listening, and it's important to be able to identify them. We might: not be listening, we might listen from habit, listen to form a response, listen with an open mind, listen with an open heart, and listen with compassion - being fully present.

Not Listening

Sometimes we have to admit we're not actually listening at all. We may think that we can look at the phone, answer emails, check the news, look at social media posts all the while carrying on a conversation. But the reality is, we really can't do all of that at the same time. Our modern life has created an erosion of our attention spans – some reports even claim that we have attention spans shorter than a goldfish!

And we have the pressure of marketers competing for our attention. In a sense, our attention is the commodity that they most covet. Recapturing our attention, and learning to not be so easily distracted for ourselves would add to our quality of life.

Listening Out of Habit

Sometimes we listen out of habit. Maybe we think we've heard the same thing so many times, we know what comes next. Maybe we're mind reading since we don't really trust that they know what they're saying, and we're going to correct their narrative. We are being disrespectful when we do this. You may have seen some of the videos on social media of nurse influencers who tease and mock the various types of nurses giving report: the confused one, the disorganized one, the too many details one, the not enough detail one, and so on. Anytime we think we can pigeon hole someone, we risk listening out of habit. This can trip us up when something new is added, or we're caught not really listening.

Listening to Form an Argument

We may have been guilty of listening in order to form an argument or other response. We're assuming that we know what they're going to say. We know we disagree, so we want to be ready with a clever retort. Or, we can't wait to share our similar experience with them, defeating their desire to share their feeling or experience with us, only to have us say, "Oh, I know exactly how you feel. That happened to me, too!"

Listening With an Open Mind

Other ways to listen, include listening with an open mind – we're willing to learn. We take in new information, asking questions to clarify and note differences. During a patient assessment, this quality is especially important. We may find that sometimes the way a patient describes their symptoms doesn't match the way we in the medical field would. You may have had a patient who denies that they have any pain, yet you can see them guarding the injured part, or grimacing when they're moved or touched. When we ask what it feels like, they may describe a "deep ache," or "like a hot poker," or "pins and needles." They don't consider it "pain," yet they do need pain management for their somatic, neurologic, or visceral pain.

Listen With an Open Heart

We can also listen with an open heart. We can see through the other person's eyes, making an emotional connection. We set aside our personal point of view for a moment in order to understand that, while their response to a situation might be different from ours, it is their truth. Our open heart helps us to recognize their feelings, and to be able to process and restate our understanding of their feelings.

Listening With Compassion

Listening with compassion means that we're fully present with the other person. We're calm and have the stability needed to be with them, even when they're in a lot of pain; even when we're feeling uncomfortable. An old habit might be to try to fix. As Brené Brown mentioned in her presentation, putting a silver lining around their pain. When that happens, it's important to take a breath, reconnect with ourselves, and recognize what's happening within us. Then we can return to listening and being present with the patient. We're willing not to have the answers or try to fix the problem, but we're partnering with them to companion them on their journey.

Respond

We want to respond instead of react. Responding with respect, being sensitive to their cues, understanding the whole person, knowing the person's priorities of care, and deciding how to best approach the situation is the goal. Every human being deserves to be treated with dignity and respect. We want that for ourselves and our patients want that as well.

Following the patient's cues is important. You've probably heard the phrase, the "COPD personality" (often said with an eye roll), but why are COPD patients sometimes impatient. They often have to manage their energy very carefully. If they get out of breath before a meal, they may not be able to eat their full meal because of being out of breath. So if you go into the room before mealtime and ask them a bunch of questions, they may very well tell you to get lost. Not being able to breathe is terrifying and they want to avoid a crisis above all else.

In order to follow our Platinum Rule, we need to understand the whole person. Each of us is more than the sum of our parts. When we take a look at their values, culture, religious practices, and family dynamics, we get a better picture of who they are as a person. Knowing the patient's priorities of care, allows us to better plan their care and discover the social determinants of health affecting them.

When we understand that, we realize that if their choices are different from ours, that's okay. We can let ourselves off the hook. They don't have to follow what we say. In fact, we're far more likely to find a solution that they can follow, when we know those priorities and preferences.

Understanding where the patient is coming from and what issues impact them, can help us respond to their needs, and sometimes demands, appropriately when we've connected first with ourselves, and then with them as an individual. Our response is a decision that will help them.

There will be times when responding with respect will be challenging. We've all had experiences with patients who were disrespectful or even combative with us. It's tough to keep that from affecting how we react to them. Taking the high road can feel less than gratifying, but in the long run, keeping our cool and living up to our values of being respectful and compassionate is worth it.

Evaluate and End

Lastly, we Evaluate and End the encounter with the patient. Were the interventions you planned effective? Did you gain the bigger picture of the patient's life? Is the plan of care individualized in a real way, and did the patient understand and have confidence in the plan? When thinking about the plan of care for the patient, does it reflect their priorities, support needs, and limitations? Will they be able to comply with the discharge plan or is the plan just wishful thinking? Do they understand what's happening? And does it make sense to them in their worldview?

Take a moment after the interaction with the patient to consider not only the medical evaluation, but your personal one as well. Were you able to use the C.A.R.E. process effectively? How did it go? Did you gain a bigger picture of the person's life? Do you feel you connected with them in a meaningful way? Did you empathize with them, even if you've never experienced what they're going through, or even if you disagree with their reactions and decisions?

When ending an interaction with a patient, leave that interaction peacefully. Even if things didn't go as well as you'd hoped, understand that all of this takes practice and there will be times that even the very best of plans and intentions won't be successful.

You may also leave with a sense that you really did connect with the patient and have a clearer understanding of them. That's something to celebrate! Wish them well and move on to the next task, giving that next interaction your full attention.

CHAPTER 5

Applied C.A.R.E.

Applying the Steps of C.A.R.E. – Case Studies

Remember the steps of C.A.R.E.: Connect, Assess, Respond, Evaluate and End as we look at some case studies.

The Bike Messenger

A young man in the emergency department had a bike accident and has an injured left hand. He's right handed, so the impairment won't be too burdensome, but he's very upset and agitated. His pain has been addressed, but he's carrying on like his life is at risk. What do you do?

Connect

Connect with yourself, take a breath and center your attention so you can be fully present with the patient. It only takes a second. Stay aware of your co-workers report and opinions, but keep an open mind as you enter the room.

How would you connect with this young man? In addition to the physical assessment, what other questions would you ask? What are the conditions would you suspect? And what personal factors might contribute to his distress? Make a note of what you'd be thinking in this case.

Assess

Assess yourself. Are there patients you find difficult to relate to? Maybe patients that seem to overreact to their condition, or who talk about everything under the sun except what's important to their care? Or who are a certain age, ethnic group, race or religion? Think about how you've worked with patients like this in the past, taking a moment to connect with yourself and assess the situation. Assure that you are staying in alignment with your values, and your intention to be compassionate.

Respond

Is it difficult for you to respond instead of reacting when patients are highly anxious? Is it easy for you to collaborate with your patient to come up with a treatment plan, or do you have a tendency to know what the plan needs to be and want to move on?

Remember that the goal is not patient compliance, but developing a plan that will work for them in their real world situation.

Evaluate and End

Would the patient feel he had told his story and was listened to? Would the patient feel empowered to have a full say in his treatment plan? Would you feel gratified that the best possible plan was created for this young man?

Well, it turns out he was a concert pianist. The young man was a student at a prestigious musical school and was preparing for his first big audition. His career might hang in the balance if he couldn't play to the best of his abilities. His anxiety was understandable in this context. Responding to him with compassion and respect, assured that he got the appropriate referrals, support, and help that he needed.

What if the patient is unresponsive?

Patients who are unresponsive, pediatric patients, and those with cognitive issues or neurodiversity can pose a challenge to our assessment skills. We can't limit our care for them to our objective observations of their physical condition. They are more than the sum of their parts, too, and uncovering what matters to them is a crucial part of compassionate care.

Remembering Maria

An elderly woman in a nursing home and also on hospice was considered disruptive because she was humming, flailing her arms around, and being uncooperative. The nursing home staff wanted to increase her anti-anxiety medication, but the hospice staff was reluctant to do so, fearing a chemical restraint.

At a joint care planning meeting, the question was asked: What did she do for a living? What were her hobbies and interests? Basically asking the question "What matters to you?" This is a question that can be asked of any patient, including children, those with cognitive issues or neurodiversity, and those who are unresponsive. But we will need to modify how we ask, and how we listen to the response.

For Maria, even though she was unresponsive, the question was still important. The family reported that she had been an opera singer. A CD player was brought to her room, and some of her favorite operatic music was played. When the arias of the world renowned Maria Callas, who she had admired, were played, her eyes lit up. She started humming along and gesturing her arms gracefully.

What had been thought of as disruptive behavior was actually her remembering her lifelong love of opera. She didn't need medication – she needed music! The staff played her music often and she always brightened up when she heard it. She died listening to the strains of the music she loved. She died peacefully.

What were the C.A.R.E. steps that were used? The nurse first connected with herself. She understood where the nursing home staff were coming from, and realized that was important. Connecting with the patient was difficult because of her unresponsiveness. In her assessment of herself, the nurse recognized her empathy with the patient. The nurse also empathized with the nursing home staff, and respectfully sought additional information.

In addition to a physical assessment of the patient, she asked questions of the patient's family. To respond, the nurse paused to consider her position. She explained her proposal professionally to the nursing home staff. She approached the patient with compassion and understanding. To evaluate and end, the nurse reviewed her use of the C.A.R.E. process and reviewed her interactions with the nursing home staff. The positive response of the patient to the opera music was a beautiful thing; a true enhancement to her quality of life.

What's Next?

Perhaps you're wondering what you should do next. I hope that you feel confident to take actions based on this process starting tomorrow. You can use the C.A.R.E. process to determine that as well.

Connect to yourself

How are you feeling about the possibility of putting compassion at the center of your work life? Do you have any trepidations about how this might be received, or are you convinced that you and your unit will benefit. I can say that in working with other nurses and organizations, even some of the skeptics found that it was needed and effective.

Assess Your Situation

Know your situation and understand your staff, including their morale, burnout, and engagement. How are their individualized plans of care and discharge plans, survey results, and their level of caring?

Be sure you know your unit situation. Do you have issues with staff morale, burnout, and incivility? We know we hate the term "nurses eat their young," and we want to be sure that that's not happening in our unit, so be sure to address this. Are the patient's care plans individualized and reflect the patient's priorities, preferences, and their social determinants of health? Do your unit survey results reflect that the staff treat all patients with respect? And are you confident that your staff provides compassionate care?

It's important to measure, even in our own informal notes and survey of charts to know how staff are doing and how they treat their patients.

Respond to What You Find

Like you, I became a nurse leader because I saw areas in my unit that needed improvement, and I knew through staff education and modeling quality care, I could make a difference. But I did find that simply telling people what to do, doesn't work. We can't just tell our staff be more compassionate.

By modeling this behavior and modeling this method, you'll be able to have a deeper understanding of how it works. When you introduce it to your staff, it will have an impact to improve how they respond to their patients, and to each other.

Evaluate and End

Looking back on how the process worked will help you evaluate the potential transformation in your and your team's life. You need to understand your own self-care and self compassion needs, what your connection with the staff is like, and your knowledge of what matters to your patients and their families. Measure the before and after for self-care and self-compassion. Try the steps of C.A.R.E., measuring the changes you see in your own attitude and satisfaction, in your interactions with your staff and co-workers, and in patient satisfaction.

When you go home after a long shift, you'll be able to tell that you've made a difference for yourself, your staff, and your patients.

CHAPTER 6

Holistic Assessment

An important part of Compassion Centered C.A.R.E. is expanding our knowledge of nursing assessment to include a holistic approach to care. In this context, holistic refers to the understanding that each of us is more than the sum of our parts. We learn in nursing school about the medical aspects of care, but sometimes other factors that impact care like psychosocial needs, cultural considerations, and the many social determinants of health are not emphasized. These factors are crucial if we are to provide compassionate care that is centered on the needs and priorities of the patient, and that look critically and realistically at the patient's reality and their world view.

I'll introduce a simple framework of doing a holistic assessment that will work for you regardless of your organization's charting system. And, we'll see how this framework will make your care and discharge plans more effective. The goal is always to help our patients by easing the burden of their suffering, and partnering with them for the best possible long term care and support. You'll find that this framework is also very satisfying for you as a nurse or other healthcare professional. By listening to our patients in an objective and nonjudgmental way, we can release the stress we sometimes feel when we believe we must give the patient the one right plan, and if that plan isn't followed, we've somehow failed. By creatively and open-heartedly, trusting our patients to know what's best for them at any given time, we treat them with respect and they feel that they can trust us. Listening builds trust, and trust builds confidence in accepting and taking our best advice. Especially, when that advice takes their needs and values into account.

More Than the Sum of Our Parts

Each person we meet is more than the sum of their parts, yet when learning about healthcare, in order to break down the enormous amount of information we need to learn, we break this knowledge down into its component parts. Any person coming to us for healthcare, has a medical condition and its associated problem list. We need to do a head to toe assessment, often breaking down the assessment into the major systems of the body. We look at the body's structure and function, but sometimes forget to incorporate the other aspects of what it means to be a human being.

Additionally, we need to bear in mind that the patient's psychosocial, spiritual, cultural, attitudes about healthcare including their past interactions with healthcare professionals and organizations, other beliefs, and how the patient wants and needs to be communicated with, affects the assessment. While we won't be the expert at all of these dimensions, it's important that we are aware of them and how they impact the patient's current condition, what their plan of care needs to include, and how to create a successful discharge plan for the patient. We also want to be aware of any risk factors that necessitate a referral to the appropriate professional in that role. Social Workers, Counselors, Board Certified Chaplains, Child Life Specialists, Therapists, and others, will be able to assist the patient and their family within their scope of practice. Don't forget to double back and review their findings. It 's important to have the full picture in mind to assure the best possible care for our patients, and the most successful discharge plan.

This graph illustrates a fuller picture of the patient. Understanding that the medical aspect of their lives are not necessarily the most dominant concern. Because we devote our lives to learning and dealing with medical conditions, we have a bias toward putting medical care first. Often patients prioritize other aspects of their lives over the medical or "taking care of themselves." The goal for healthcare really isn't "compliance," even though we have a hard time letting that idea go. Our goal is actually to help find the plan of care that includes all aspects of the patient's world view, promotes trust in the healthcare professionals on their team, and enhances communication between all these individuals.

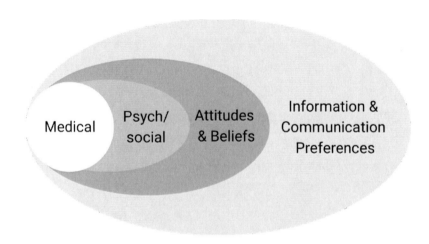

International Classification of Functioning, Disability, and Health

The World Health Organization has created an International Classification of Functioning, Disability, and Health – also known as the ICF. The ICF is an important innovation in the way we look at disability. It standardizes the characterization of structural and functional impairments, and relates them to a patient's activity limitations and participation restrictions. It goes further by looking closely at the support a patient needs, and correlates those needs with the resources available within the context of their environment and world view.

Components of the ICF:

- ❖ Functioning and disability
  - ✓ Body functions and structures
  - ✓ Includes psychosocial, emotional, mental illness, and family dynamics
  - ✓ Activities and participation
- ❖ Contextual Factors
  - ✓ Environmental factors
  - ✓ Personal factors

This grid illustrates the dimensions of a health condition, connecting the factors involved. You can see that this grid places "activities" at the center of the patient's health

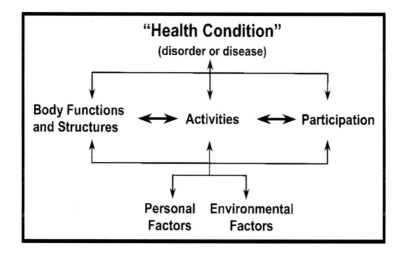

condition. This helps us see that disability is actually a continuum and where the patient falls on that continuum can change, and will certainly be affected by the levels of support available to them.

The contextual factors involved in the patient's support include environmental factors made up of the physical, social, emotional, and cultural world of the patient. These contextual factors include: products and technology, support and relationships, attitudes and culture, services systems and policies.

- ❖ Environmental factors make up the physical, social, emotional, and cultural world of the patient
  - Products and technology
  - Support and relationships
  - Attitudes and culture
  - Services, systems, and policies

It is a sad fact of life that not all people have the same access to support for their medical needs. It's important for each of us to not only be aware of these healthcare inequities, but to look for ways to even the playing field for our patients. Systemic racism, sexism, ageism, and ableism can seem invisible to those of us unaffected by these systemic inequities.

We need to make a commitment to ourselves to educate ourselves on these issues, and to interrogate our assumptions about our patients, and understand what hurdles they must overcome. By understanding these issues, listening to and believing our patients when they express their frustrations with these problems, and not being afraid to recognize our role in these systems is crucial.

Keeping an open mind, and keeping an eagle eye out for these issues can help us be proactive in helping our patients overcoming these hurdles. We want to be part of the solution for our patients, not part of the problem!

CHAPTER 7

The Basics of Assessment

Structure and function is the most common approach to assessment. We're all familiar with the assessment checklist that focuses on structure, function, and symptoms. For the most part, this part of the assessment is easy and straightforward. We can use our four senses to assess: touch and palpation, listening to heart and other internal sounds, observing the external structures and movement, and even smell in the case of wound infections. We use diagnostic methods to assess the patient's systems and function. X-rays and scans, lab results, monitoring, and other methods enhance and confirm our assessments.

Structure and Function

❖ Is the structure sound?

❖ Does everything function?

❖ Are there structural impairments?

❖ Are there functional limitations?

❖ What are the patient's symptoms?

Becoming not only competent but expert at assessment is a major goal for all healthcare professionals. Then it's important to broaden our horizons to include all of the dimensions of a person and their world view.

Impairments

❖ Problems in body function or structure such as significant deviation or loss:

✓ Mental functions

✓ Sensory functions and pain

✓ Functions of body systems

Once we assess and understand the patient's problems with the structure and function of their bodily systems, the next step is to understand the limitations these problems place on the patient. The patient will be affected by the patient's mental functions, their sensory functions and pain, and the functions of their body systems.

Many factors enter into the patient's perception of their health problems. A patient who has been lucky and has never been ill or had a major injury before, may be quite shocked at their condition. They may have been less than empathetic with others who have illness or injury because they had no frame of reference; it's hard to believe that this "hurts so much!" or they may become very worried or even obsessed with what will happen next. "How could this happen to me?" might be something you'll hear these kinds of patients say. Patients who have been "health nuts" and feel they did everything right, may feel that their medical problem can't be true.

On the other hand, you may have patients who have had chronic illnesses or disabilities for a long time; even for most of their lives. They may feel that they have had to fight with the healthcare system to get what they need. They've heard all the questions, and can be quite weary of hearing the same questions – sometimes multiple times a day! They can also feel that healthcare professionals are judging or even blaming them for their condition. Mainly, they don't understand why we don't listen to them.

Subjective Symptoms

Pain and other symptoms are affected by these factors as well. Something that is very important to understand is that pain or other symptom scales are simply a way for the patient to compare their perception of pain or other symptoms. Pain is always subjective. The pain scale does not turn a subjective experience into an objective observation. It's important to recognize that the pain score is NOT a dosing guide. When a pain naïve patient reports that their pain is on the severe end of the scale, that report does not mean that we abandon good pain management principles. We still "start low and go slow," and have close and consistent evaluation of the patient's pain. A patient who has had chronic pain for years might report their pain at 4 with a goal of 2, but the medication type and dosage might be what we'd expect only for someone in severe pain. The reality is that, if we could experience that patient's pain, we'd probably be knocked to our knees!

Also important to realize that a patient's perception of their pain is strongly affected by their emotional state. If they feel very emotional, perhaps they are going through a personal trauma like a divorce, or being estranged from their family, or feeling spiritual despair, they may report their pain being very intense. Again, we start low and go slow with their pain medication, but when there are emotional, spiritual, or psychological issues compounding the situation, we won't be able to get their pain under control without addressing these issues. A consult with the Social Worker, Licensed Mental Health Counselor, or Board Certified Chaplain may go a long way in helping the patient.

Another patient might feel that they're being a burden on us, or that they are weak if they admit that they have pain. We need to observe if they are guarding the part that is affected, their facial expression, tone of voice, ability to ambulate, appetite, quality of sleep, and others clues that show that they are experiencing pain. Helping them to voice their concerns, perhaps bringing in the Social Worker to ask the "why" question, can help in understanding and working with the underlying problems to find a way to palliate the patient's pain. This will enhance the patient's over-all wellness and quality of life.

The most important thing to remember is that we must use our professional knowledge of care and treatment, and to include the complexities of how our patients perceive their condition. Just because we've observed a procedure many times, and might even believe that it doesn't really hurt that much, or it's really not a big deal, that doesn't mean that the patient has that kind of confidence in what's happening to them. They can be terrified by what we consider routine.

Activity Limitations

Limitations are what is most important to our patients. When a patient has physical structural, functional, or symptom problems, the limitations this places on the patient's life is at the forefront of the patient's mind.

Limitations
- ❖ Activity limitations
- ❖ Participation restrictions
    - ✓ Mobility
    - ✓ Self-care
    - ✓ Relationships and interactions
    - ✓ Community and social life

A simple example would be a patient who has a broken arm. If the left arm is broken, and the patient is right handed, the limitation is less than if the dominant arm is affected. You can probably think of more examples along this line. Someone who works in an office environment, may be able to use a voice activated system on their computer so they can continue their work with only minor inconvenience. On the other hand, if a construction worker breaks their arm, they may be out of work for weeks as the break heals. Or, they may choose to continue to work, but be really hard on the cast, and not follow the recommendations for limiting the range of motion in the associated joints.

All of us have important activities that we need to continue to stay healthy and survive, and to enjoy our lives. Mobility and self-care are important for all of us. For our patients, limitations on their basic activities of daily living and self-care can be factors that either allow the patient to recover, or that will lead to decline in the patient's condition, maybe even creating a life limiting situation.

Part of what makes life worth living is our ability to interact with others and create healthy relationships. We thrive when we have these individual relationships, and can interact with our community, and have an active social life. When these relationships are limited, our health can suffer even further.

This chart gives an example of a scale that could be used to evaluate a patient's limitations. When we can measure the patient's limitations based on their individual circumstances, we can look at ways we can support them. We can also use a chart like this to evaluate the plan of care and treatments provided. There will be situations when the patient's limitations won't be possible to improve due to their disability. However, this does not mean that we have no further care to provide. We continue to be creative in looking for ways to mitigate the patient's perceptions of their limitations, ways to bring other aspects of their life to the forefront, and how to use technology, durable medical equipment, or social support to meet the patient's needs.

Level	Description	Qualifiers
0	None	No limitations
1	Mild	Present < 25% of the time, tolerable, happened rarely over the last 30 days
2	Moderate	Present < 50% of the time, interfering with day to day life, happened occasionally over the last 30 days
3	Severe	Present > 50% of the time, partially disrupting day to day life, happened frequently over the last 30 days
4	Complete	Present > 95% of the time, totally disrupting day to day life, happened every day over the last 30 days

For example, a young man who had progressive muscular degeneration felt socially isolated and very lonely. By providing him with a laptop computer, he was able to enter a community college system and take online classes that included real time class discussions. There were online social games and forums he participated in with good success. While it wasn't possible for him to travel often, he was able to be transported to the college for the end of his favorite class using an electric wheelchair to attend with his classmates and connect in person. Appropriate support made all the difference.

Contextual Factors

I'm sure the role of contextual factors in the patient's condition is becoming clear. When a patient is in our environment, we can forget that the limitations in their environment can have a big impact.

Contextual Factors

❖ Environmental factors make up the physical, social, emotional, and cultural world of the patient

- Products and technology
- Support and relationships
- Attitudes and culture
- Services, systems, and policies

The patient's environmental factors make up the physical, social, emotional, and cultural world of the patient can include: products and technology, support and relationships, attitudes and culture, and services, systems, and policies. We looked at the over-view of these points, so let's look at a few examples of how these might affect individual patients.

We mentioned the young man who was able to utilize a computer with network capabilities and a motorized wheelchair to enhance his quality of life, and there are many more examples. The patient's family, community, religion, culture, and other societal factors can make a big difference in a patient's condition, progress, and healing efforts. When a patient's plan of care includes medications that are not part of their insurance policy's formulary, and the patient cannot afford the medication, they will not be able to take that medication. Rather than judging them "non-compliant," we can look closer to find other medica tions or provide help in appealing insurance company decisions. For patients without insurance, this becomes even more important and challenging for the team to respond to.

World View

The patient's family, culture, religious, and social rules and norms can make a big difference as well. A patient may believe in the cultural remedies of their family and ancestors. They may value these remedies more than the medical care we recommend. They might even hide their desire to use these traditions if they feel we will be judgmental or forbid them. By being open to their beliefs, we can assure that our plan of care accommodates these remedies, assuring there are no adverse interactions, or looking at the timing of medications and procedures. This will assure that the patient retains the support of their family and community, and illustrates our respect for dignity in their identity.

On the other hand, the patient's identity may be in conflict with their family and culture or religion. For example, a transgender patient may be rejected by their family and be considered as going against strongly held religious beliefs. They may find themselves homeless or searching for a sympathetic community for support. When working with this patient, sensitivity is important. We need to assure that we use their preferred name and pronouns, and that we give extra care during a physical exam for privacy and consent. You may have noticed the use of "they" and "their" in the singular in this book. While that is not a common usage for many, it is correct and helps in emphasizing inclusion. In fact, in some organizations, it is common to see all staff's preferred pronouns on their name badge. This helps normalize asking for and using this information appropriately.

Patients might be part of a culture where the gendered rules are very strict for who makes decisions about the healthcare of the members of a family. The head of the household, often the elder male of the family might insist on making final decisions about care, medication, or other treatments. He might even dictate what can and cannot be shared with the patient about their condition. This can be common in end of life cases, and hospices often find families who want to shield their loved ones from the reality of their prognosis. Each healthcare professional must come to terms with these situations, which can fly in the face of our modern sensibilities about informed consent, veracity, and decision making. It can be difficult, but it is important to approach these situations with an open mind, looking for alternatives that will satisfy the root cause of the patients needs.

Peace of Mind

Even when a patient's culture goes against our strongly held beliefs, we must make an effort to interrogate our beliefs to find a way to accept the patient and their family in a way that is respectful of their dignity. We don't have to agree or join practices that we disagree with, but as long as it is not harming the patient, they have the right to their beliefs and practices. Our job is to support them in the best way we can. We can develop a sense of calmness and composure – equanimity – that will give us peace of mind.

Quality of Life

This chart, from the Centers for Disease Control and Prevention provides additional clarity on how the contextual factors affect the patient's disease progression as well as the place of contextual factors in the hierarchy of healthcare.

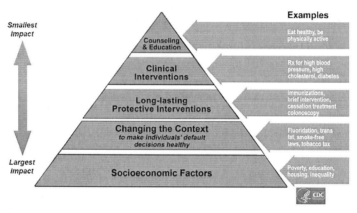

Adapted from Thomas R. Frieden. A Framework for Public Health Action: The Health Impact Pyramid. American Journal of Public Health: April 2010, Vol. 100, No. 4, pp. 590-595. doi: 10.2105/AJPH.2009.185652

You'll see that the socioeconomic factors are considered as having the largest impact on factors that affect health. We often think of our lifestyle choices to be the most important drivers in health, but this just isn't the case. While lifestyle can certainly help with quality of life, and there are risk factors involved, those factors are far less impactful than the patient's socioeconomic factors, systemic issues, equity disparity, and availability of protective interventions.

We'd love to believe that if we can just do everything right with our health, we'll be spared unpleasant conditions and diseases. You may have heard people say that if they eat a vegan diet, never smoke, or keep to a special (often expensive) diet or supplements, etc., they will be bulletproof and never get sick. The reality is that patients who have never smoked or even been around smokers can develop lung cancer, and there are smokers who never develop respiratory illness. The fact of the matter is that many of these diseases are too complex to be able to chalk up to lifestyle choices that contribute less to the outcome than we might think.

Of course we want to encourage our patients to develop good habits and lifestyle choices that will enhance their quality of life. But we do need to be cautious that we don't wind up shaming our patients or blaming them for their condition.

Support

Support and connection are crucial for patients to heal and thrive. When a patient has limitations, finding and cultivating interpersonal support is so important. This support includes: self-care, relationships and interactions, community and social life, mobility, and financial support.

Support Factors

❖ What support is needed for the patient's limitations?

  ✓ Self-care

  ✓ Relationships & interactions

  ✓ Community & social life

  ✓ Mobility

  ✓ Financial

Self-care can include things like finding time to do something fun or special like going to a movie or out to dinner, to the more in-depth care like prayer life and philosophical contemplation. In our relationships, we need connections with people who we can trust to have conversations with that share our inner most thoughts, fears, and concerns. These relationships can vary depending on the history between the individuals. In each of these, forming and maintaining healthy boundaries is a key area that will protect the relationships and the patient's well-being.

Community and social life is important to some patients. A person who is used to being involved in social, cultural, or religious groups, perhaps even being a leader in the organization may feel real grief when these activities are curtailed due to illness. As illness progresses, the role of the patient will shift and change in the family or social settings.

A man who has been the head of household, perhaps a leader in his work or community, may grieve the loss of his role when others in the family need to step in and take charge in many situations. In a family where mom has always taken care of everyone in the family, and has always been the one who always brings the best casserole to the pot luck, may find that members of the family and group are at a loss for how to care for her.

In any of these cases, it's important that we identify potential problems and work with the family to find solutions that may include bringing in outside caregivers, training for the family or friends, or other ways the patient's needs can be met within the context of the family situation.

CHAPTER 8

The Next Level

We can take assessment to the next level by recognizing that our observations need to include the factors that personalize the patient's priorities and life. When we assess any patient, when we've determined their structure and function, it's important to then ask questions about their limitations. Some of the questions we need to ask include:

- ✓ How does the patient respond to their limitations?
- ✓ How do they respond to the treatment for their problem?
- ✓ Are they being optimally treated?
- ✓ What resources are available to the patients?

Assessment Framework

Inspired by the WHO's ICF, this is a framework for assessment that includes the holistic factors that see the patient as a full person. Whether in the physical, psychosocial, or spiritual/cultural dimensions, we can assess by going through each aspect of the patient: structure, function, limitations, and support. Let's go through an example for physical problems first.

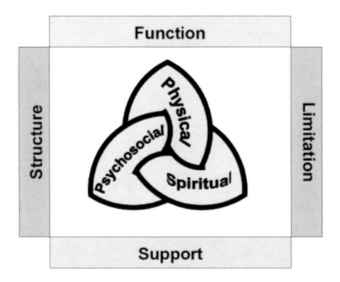

Structure

In looking at the patient's physical structure, we do a head-to-toe assessment using basic anatomy and physical systems. We may use a charting checklist to guide us.

Physical Structure:

- ✓ Head-to-Toe assessment
- ✓ Basic anatomy
- ✓ Physical systems
- ✓ Charting checklists

Function

Function is sometimes difficult to distinguish from the physical structure, and sometimes they are blended on your charting checklist. But think of function in terms of what the physical structure does in the body. Among these functions will be mobility issues, the pathophysiology of the disease process, and is measured with diagnostic test results, vital signs, and patient reported symptoms. Be sure to compare any of these results and measures over time. A single number isn't as meaningful to understanding the patient's condition as a continuum of their symptoms and other measures.

Physical Function:
- ✓ Mobility issues
- ✓ Pathophysiology
- ✓ Diagnostic test results
- ✓ Vital signs
- ✓ Compare results over time

Limitations

Understanding the limitations a condition has on a patient is key to developing an individualized plan of care. We discussed some possible scenarios where limitations can be a strong factor for the patient. During the assessment and throughout the patient's stay, an ongoing assessment will help your understanding of the patient's world view.

Be sure to ask about their symptoms, mobility issues, systemic limitations, and their understanding of their role or employment, the emotional impact of their illness, and their quality of life.

Physical Limitations:

- ✓ Symptoms
- ✓ Mobility issues
- ✓ Systemic limitations
- ✓ Patient reporting:

  - Role or employment

  - Emotional impact

  - Quality of life

Support

By looking at the support the patient needs, a discharge plan can be developed that will have a far greater chance of success for the patient than creating a plan that is a cookie cutter approach. When we take all of these factors into consideration, the patient will feel heard, and will be an active participant in their on-going healthcare.

Don't make assumptions – review with the patient what resources they have, and what they will need. This is an important time to take an interdisciplinary approach. If the case is complicated, the facility social worker will be able to make community connections for the patient to help with financial, social, and referral needs.

Physical Support:

- ✓ What support do they have?
- ✓ What support do they need?
  - Financial
  - Healthcare availability
  - Family help
  - Assistive devices
  - Medication

Patients do not respond as well when they have treatment plans dictated to them. In a holistic, patient-centered approach, the patient is an active participant in their care. We need to listen to what matters to them, what aspects affect the plan of care, and how the team can work together to come up with creative solutions that will be successful.

Nothing about me, without me

Dimensions of Life

We reviewed using the holistic assessment framework for the physical assessment, now let's take a look at using it with other dimensions of the patient's life. In the psycho-social dimension of the patient, we can look at a variety of aspects. Their emotional life, social and community life, and their relationship within their family unit.

Family Structure

When assessing the family, start with the structure of the family. Find out who the members of the family are, and if anyone is missing. Remember that not all families have a traditional structure: they may have a blended family, be in a homosexual relationship, or have other configurations of members. A family tree, or genome, can be used to identify the members of a family, including their extended family. A genogram may be valuable to develop, and you may want to include the Social Worker or Board Certified Chaplain to help in it's development, especially if there is a complicated or particularly problematic family dynamic.

Family Structure:
- ✓ Who are they?
- ✓ Family tree
- ✓ Is anyone "missing?"
- ✓ Do they feel complete?

THE NEXT LEVEL • 91

Family Function

The function of the members of the family, and the family as a whole unit are varied and complex. A major aspect to consider are the roles of the members of the family. It is very important for the healthcare professional to be non-judgmental about the family structure and the roles within the family. If the family is unconventional, don't assume that it is dysfunctional. Look at the functions of the family members as objectively as possible.

We want to assess the roles of the family members, their identity as a family, or their place in society or cultural milieu. What are the responsibilities of the family members? This may play an important role if one of the members cannot fulfil their role, and another member must step in. Families often have expectations of each other, or their social circle or culture may have expectations of them to continue being considered part of the group.

Family Function:
- ✓ What are their roles?
- ✓ What is their identity as a family?
- ✓ Responsibilities?
- ✓ Expectations?

Limitations of the Family

Look at the limitations present in the family structure, if any. For some patients, especially those with chronic disabilities, there may be tensions in the family, both with caregiver fatigue, and with issues around the ongoing care of the patient. For example, an older man with chronic COPD who still smokes, may find that his wife is very resentful that he is not taking care of himself in her eyes. She may resist fully participating in his care, or forbid that he smoke again. This might lead him to hide his smoking, putting himself and his family at risk of fire if he smokes without turning off his oxygen concentrator.

Understanding the factors that cause the limitations is important. What is causing friction among family members? What problems are they experiencing? Are there other difficulties that will make caring for the patient difficult? And what are their needs? Often the family issues are a greater problem for patient discharge planning than the patient themselves.

Family Limitations:
- ✓ What factors cause limitations?
- ✓ Friction?
- ✓ Problems?
- ✓ Other difficulties?
- ✓ What are their needs?

Family Support

The patient's immediate family is an important source of support and help, but be sure to look past the immediate family to their extended family unit, friends, social community, faith community, etc. The patient may have access to additional resources, such as online support groups, searching for additional or alternative treatments, as well as organizations specializing in their condition.

Looking at the support they have, what their over-all needs are, and look for ways to fill the gaps so that the discharge plan has the best chance of on-going success.

Family Support:
- ✓ Other family?
- ✓ Social structure?
- ✓ Faith community?
- ✓ Financial?
- ✓ Technological?
- ✓ Access to resources?

Dimensions of Life

Each person has a variety of dimensions that are worthy of being assessed. The more complete our holistic assessment is, the better chance we have for success in developing a healthcare plan that they can live with. By understanding how these aspects work together and how interconnected they are, we will have a far more complete picture of the patient. We come into the patient interaction as the "content expert," but the patient is the "life expert."

We need to give our patients our best advice, knowledge about their condition, and information about treatment options. We are an important part of the team, but we are only one member of the team. The patient must be the team leader, so that they can live their best life. We need to have patience with this approach, because the patient's decisions might not be what we would choose, or what we think is best. However, when we can show the patient that they can trust us, that we will support them and continue to contribute toward their health and well-being, they may well begin to make thoughtful movement toward wellness.

Each dimension can be approached in this format:

- ❖ Spiritual
- ❖ Cultural
- ❖ Social
- ❖ Emotional

We can ask "What matters to you?" of each patient to start the dialogue. From the simplest preference, like wanting to have their bath in the evening instead of the morning, to the more complex understanding of the impact of family and cultural dynamics on their overall healthcare;

understanding the person will allow us to give them the best possible care. A goal all healthcare professionals share.

We want to know: "What do I need to know about you as a person, to give you the best possible care?"

CHAPTER 9

Conclusion

Nurses are compassionate people, and we want to help others – we're altruistic. Yet, it can be difficult to help others when our actions aren't appreciated by some of our patients. We may have grown up in a culture where holding a person's hand and making eye contact communicated our caring. Taking over with the solution to the person's problem, telling them not to worry, and giving them instructions for what to do is a prevailing mind-set for how to provide care.

But in a pluralistic society, we might feel shocked or insulted when our efforts to provide compassionate care are rebuffed or are considered offensive. We may have learned about different cultures in school or in-service education; even considering ourselves culturally competent. Yet, the truth is that all cultures are internally diverse, and generalities are not going to help much when working with individuals.

We also work with a variety of people in our organizations. We often feel the sting of not being treated with respect by those organizations, and are frustrated with the healthcare system – a system that seems too huge to be able to change. We might hear about the importance of self-care; resilience, taking yoga classes, having "me time," and many more tools. Those things can certainly be helpful, and we should do the things that serve us. We cannot, though, fix the healthcare system by taking a yoga class.

What we can do, and what we owe ourselves, is have compassion for ourselves. Only you can know what the best course is for yourself if you're feeling burned-out, or experiencing empathic distress, or even moral injury. It could be that you need a change, and there are many avenues in healthcare that you can pursue. Nurses have many skills that are valuable in other fields as well.

You might want to stay in your current role, and be willing to take on some steps to make things better on your unit. If you are a nurse leader, you can look for ways to be the best leader you can be. It's often said, and studies show, that staff don't leave the organization, they leave their manager. We've all worked for toxic managers, yet if we asked those managers why they do the things they do, they may well feel that they have no choice; that the system is dictating how they manage.

Can you turn things around? Realistically, you will have to manage under the constraints of the system. There are things you can do to make your unit's environment far more acceptable to work in. By asking you staff "What matters to you?" listening to the answers, and doing what you can to follow up on making things better, you'll go a long way toward returning the pride and even joy in work. When people are proud of the work they are doing, they go home tired for sure, but proud to make a difference.

By centering compassion in everything we do, we don't treat anyone as expendable or merely a means to an end. Each person on the healthcare team is a valuable member deserving of compassion, respect, and dignity. The patients we serve are not just room numbers and disease processes. They have full lives that include many priorities that might not center on their medical condition.

In all of this, using the C.A.R.E. process will clarify and simplify what to do in any given situation. In Compassion Centered C.A.R.E., we see the whole person and, while we might not always agree with their decisions, we can accept their choices as right for them in that moment. Compassion also gives us hope that when the person feels that we respect them, wish the best for them, and are doing our best to help them, that they can trust us. They might even decide that we've earned their trust, and they may be more willing to try our advice, especially when it's crafted to fit with their lifestyle, contingencies, and values.

What's Next?

If you are a front line nurse leader, it's important that you know your situation:

- ✓ Are your staff's patient plans of care individualized?
- ✓ Does your staff understand their patient's social determinants of health?
- ✓ Are the patient's priorities and preferences respected and part of the plan of care and discharge plan?

Knowing where the knowledge gaps are will help in your efforts for education and training. Many times staff will complain about individualized plans of care, considering them "too hard," or not understanding how the plan can be individualized. They wonder, "Aren't all gall bladder surgeries the same?" not realizing that the differences in response to a surgery, treatment, or medication is only a small part of what makes the plan specific to the patient.

Staff may need additional education and training about the social determinants of health. Learning about how the systemic, social, and socioeconomic factors impact their patients helps staff know what questions to ask, and understanding that it's really not the patient's fault that they have difficulties following the discharge plan. They may be surprised to know that the lifestyle advice we love to give our patients might not have nearly the impact we wish they had.

But most important in this framework is the understanding of the patient's priorities and preferences. The patient is a partner in care, and compliance isn't necessarily the ultimate goal, while developing trust, treating the patient with respect, and honoring their culture and world view definitely is. The discharge plan is a crucial part of patient care. Only when we look at our patients as the team leader of their care, and see the big picture of their life will we be able to create a plan that will be successful and bring about the outcomes we hope for.

When we put this framework into action, we will see improvements in our care. Use these assessment prompts to evaluate:

- ✓ Seeing the patient as a person and a partner in care
- ✓ Improved individualized plans of care and discharge planning
- ✓ Improved patient satisfaction, reduced readmission rates, and improved compliance

Celebrate your success! Your patients will feel respected, will make better choices, and have improved outcomes.

Bibliography

Agency for Healthcare Research and Quality. (2018). CAHPS Clinician and Group Survey Measures. Rockville, MD. http://www.ahrq.gov/cahps/surveys-guidance/cg/about/survey-measures.html

Barnes-Neff, Cheryl. (2021). CARE: Connect, Assess, Respond, Evaluate. *CLOSLER Lifelong Learning in Clinical Excellence*. https://closler.org/lifelong-learning-in-clinical-excellence/3-priorities-in-palliative-care

Baughan, J. and Smith, A. (2013). *Compassion, Caring, and Communication*. New York, NY: Routledge, Taylor Francis Group.

Brown, Brené. (2013) Brené Brown on Empathy. *The RSA Org*. https://youtu.be/1Evwgu369Jw

Dignity in Care. (2016). Dignity in Care Toolkit. http://www.dignityincare.ca/en/toolkit.html

Dudgeon, K. (2015). Understanding the Whole Patient: A Model for Holistic Care. *Continuum Innovation*. Retrieved online on 4/28/2019: https://www.continuuminnovation.com/en/how-we-think/blog/understanding-the-whole-patient/

Erickson, M., Sandor, K. (Revised 2017). Core Essentials for the Practice of Holistic Nursing *The American Holistic Nurses Credentialing Corporation*.

Fogarty, RX. (2020). #DearNurses. *Dear World.org*. https://nurses.dearworld.org/013-I-ve-Never-Cried-Like-That-About-A-Patient-1

Grassman, Deborah. (2019). Anchoring Heart Technique. *Opus Peace Soul Inquiry*. https://opuspeace.org/soul-injury-inventory/soul-restoring-resources/anchoring-heart/

Guo, Q., et al. (2017). Development and Evaluation of the Dignity Talk Question Framework for Palliative Patients and Their Families. *Palliative Medicine*, Vol. 32(1) 195-205.

Halifax, Joan. (2018). *Standing at the Edge: Finding Wisdom Where Fear and Courage Meet.* New York, NY: Flatiron Books.

Institute for Healthcare Improvement. (2019). What Matters Information Page. Retrieved online on 4/29/2019: http://www.ihi.org/Topics/WhatMatters/Pages/default.aspx

Lee, Thomas. (2016). *An Epidemic of Empathy in Healthcare: How to Deliver Compassionate, Connected Patient Care That Creates a Competitive Advantage.* New York, NY: McGraw-Hill Education.

Luxford, K. (2015). Rising to the Challenge of Patient-Centered Care. *Health Management: The Journal.* Volume 15, Issue 3.

Mapping Therapy Goals to the International Classification of Functioning, Disability, and Health. (2019). *Centers for Medicare and Medicaid Services.* Retrieved online on 4/29/2019: https://www.cms.gov/Medicare/Billing/TherapyServices/Downloads/Mapping_Therapy_Goals_ICF.pdf

Ozcan, T. (2018). Can We Evaluate and Treat the Patient as a Whole? *Health Management: The Journal.* Volume 18, Issue 6. 448-450.

Perlo J, Balik B, Swensen S, Kabcenell A, Landsman J, Feeley D. (2017). IHI Framework for Improving Joy in Work: IHI White Paper. *Institute for Healthcare Improvement.* http://www.ihi.org/resources/Pages/IHIWhitePapers/Framework-Improving-Joy-in-Work.aspx

Price, R.A. et al. (2018). Development of Valid and Reliable Measures of Patient and Family Experiences of Hospice Care for Public Reporting. *Journal of Palliative Medicine*, Volume XX, Number XX.

Prodinger, B., Rastall, P., Wooldridge, D., & Carpenter, I. (2018). Documenting Routinely What Matters to People: Standardized Headings for Health Records of Patients with Chronic Health Conditions. *Applied Clinical Informatics*. Volume 9, No. 2/2018.

Rogers, Fred. (2018). Mr. Rogers' Neighborhood. https://www.misterrogers.org/

Seppälä, Emma. (2020). Social Connection Boosts Health, Even When You're Isolated, Social connection is Key to Health and Happiness. *Psychology Today.* https://www.psychologytoday.com/us/blog/feeling-it/202003/social-connection-boosts-health-even-when-youre-isolated

Trzeciak, S. and Mazzarelli, A. (2019). *Compassionomics: The Revolutionary Scientific Evidence That Caring Makes a Difference.* Pensacola, FL: Studer Group Publishing.

Weisman, Theresa. (1996). A Concept Analysis of Empathy. *Journal of Advanced Nursing.* 23, 1162-1167.

What is a Holistic Health Assessment? (2019). Lamar University, Beaumont, TX. Retrieved online on: 4/29/2019: https://degree.lamar.edu/articles/nursing/holistic-health-assessment.aspx

World Health Organization. International Classification of Functioning, Disability, and Health. Information page, updated 2 March 2018. Retrieved on 4/29/2019: https://www.who.int/classifications/icf/en/

Zamanzadeh, V, Jasemi, M, Valizadeh, L, Koegh, B., & Taleghani, F. (2015). Effective Factors in Providing Holistic Care: A Qualitative Study. *Indian Journal of Palliative Care.* 21(2). 214-224.

Acknowledgements

There are many people to acknowledge and thank. I want to thank my editor, and the wonderful people at Laurel Oak Press for their help and support. I'd like to thank Sarah Cordiner, author and course creation specialist, who helped guide the creation of this book. There have been many mentors along the way, and I'd like to thank Sylvia Parker my nurse mentor when I began working in hospice for helping me understand a more holistic way to see my patients, Carmen Demos and Jillian Madsen for honing my work on the holistic conceptual framework, and the many nurses who listened to my talks and classes, and gave me invaluable feedback and encouragement.

I would also like to acknowledge and thank my family. My son Chris and partner Matt have been such a strong support throughout this adventure in creating courses and this book. Even though they have had to put up with my late nights, helping me through frustrations with the computer, and listening to me go on and on about some new idea or concept, they were always there for me.

Lastly, I must thank my bestie and mother-in-law, Carol Foster without whom this book would not exist. Through her own adventures in writing, I have learned a lot about editing, book publishing, book design – we have learned together, and I look forward to more fun with books!

About the Author

Cheryl Barnes-Neff has been a Registered Nurse for over forty years, with decades of management and quality improvement experience. Having worked in a variety of healthcare settings from neo-natal intensive care to hospice care, she developed an understanding for the importance of quality nursing care. With a commitment to lifelong learning, she has earned a number of certifications, two Master's degrees, and a Doctorate.

Always interested in culture and religion, she has immersing herself in both through learning and travel. This interest has enabled her to integrate patient care in not only the physical, but the psychosocial, spiritual, and cultural dimensions. She found her calling in hospice care, and has spent over twenty years as a hospice nurse, educator, quality manager, and chaplain.

During her career, she's seen many patient care models come and go: From team nursing, to primary care, to care management, all the way to today's most popular model, patient centered care. None of those models takes a holistic view of healthcare, and her proposal is that our care model should actually be Compassion Centered C.A.R.E. With compassion in the center, we're applying compassion to ourselves, our co-workers, and to our patients and their families.

For More Information

For more information about Compassion Centered C.A.R.E., please visit *barnesneff.com* to read additional articles about compassion, care, and nursing leadership.

Continuing education courses are available, including free one hour credit courses on the *Introduction to Compassion Centered C.A.R.E.* and *Holistic Assessment*. An in depth workshop *C.A.R.E. About What Matters* is also available to take a deeper dive into how to apply these important concepts.

Enroll in our learning portal to find out more and sign up for classes at https://courses.barnesneff.com/

Connect with me on Social Media at:

LinkedIn
https://www.linkedin.com/in/cheryl-barnes-neff/

Instagram
https://www.instagram.com/cheryl.barnes_neff/

Twitter
https://twitter.com/BarnesNeff

Facebook
https://www.facebook.com/authorcherylbarnesneff

NOTES

NOTES

Made in United States
North Haven, CT
12 July 2024

54717605R00071